I TRIED, I FAILED, BUT

I STAYED STRONG

TE-AI INTREBAT VREO-
DATĂ CUM E SĂ SLĂBEȘ-
TI 11 KILOGRAME INTR-O
SĂPTĂMÂNĂ? EROUL CĂRȚII
DE FAȚĂ E UN TÂNĂR CARE A
REUSIT ACEASTĂ PERFOR-
MANȚĂ PENTRU A PARTICIPA
LA O COMPETIȚIE SPORTIVĂ!

AMIR JOY

ISBN: 978-1-7088558-6-4

For more information, visit:
www.amirjoy.net

DEDICATION:

Dedicated to FREE MYSELF

CONTENTS

SUPPORT
THE AUTHOR:

I self-publish privately, therefore, anyone, if interested, can support me and check out my services on my website:

www.amirjoy.net

"When the going gets tough, put one foot in
front of the other and just keep going. Don't give up."
(Roy T. Bennett, The Light in the Heart)

PREFACE:

My esteemed reader, I have no notion why I have written this book. Perhaps I have written it for sharing my journey amongst you. Perhaps for relieving myself from the distress which I have faced. Perhaps for showing people that losing weight isn't as easy as some think. Perhaps to give those who seek to lose weight but aren't motivated enough a push to get started. Either way, perhaps one day I may know…

All the things you are about to read are precisely detailed for during each of the mentioned days, I would take physical and mental notes of what had occurred during that day. The journey is filled with mixed emotions, chiefly despair and suffering. I know the book is about losing those 25lbs (11kgs), but I have tried to write the book as a story, narrating each chapter as a day. The pounds I have lost were due to a competition I had to compete in. Thus, I wouldn't have even tried to attempt the act without a valid reason. Throughout this book, you will be able to feel my emotions. During the journey I'm about to disclose, I have written some accounts that are, more or less, like a diary of what was going through my mind at the time. I'll quote them throughout the journey for you to get the feeling of the situation more precisely. But, before you, my esteemed reader, start the journey, I need to lay on the surface some facts or an account that would set you on the page in life I am currently at. These details will help you grasp my situation or state of mind at the time quite better. Possibly, even share the exact feelings and emotions I had. I'll keep a long story short, therefore, without keeping you any longer, I say we commence with my brief account.

Here's a classic/cliché situation for you. Ever had a dream or a goal and the people around you, most probably the closest, would rip it down? Telling you to leave all the bollocks you've been training and working hard for and start focusing on what's important. A legit career. Telling you "all you're doing is wasting your time". Telling you, "it wouldn't get you anywhere." Saying that it's child's play, a joke. And the hardest part is when, no matter your achievements or talents, they still won't view them as genuine—ripping your dream apart. Yes indeed, that's what I'm stuck myself into.

My father was/still is a businessman. He has his business that, arguably, takes up his life. Like father like son, he hoped I would take up his business someday. Now, before I got involved in boxing, I was playing football/soccer for a football club in my city. Football to me was like dopamine to an addict.

I played football most of my life when, unfortunately, injuries came into play. I had a groin strain on both legs—a complete tear. I couldn't play anymore. Treatments weren't having their desired effect. My legs wouldn't heal. My limit was 1 game per week. The days after the game, the pain from both legs wouldn't let me train or even run. I had to wait a couple of days for them to heal. I was shattered. I didn't know what to do anymore.

By that time, I was about 15. I started going to my father's workplace, for I faced reality. No more sprinting, thus no more football. I assume my father was the most delighted one with my going to his workplace and learning the family business. I know my father wouldn't care. That's just his personality. His business is his life. He worked from poverty since he was 14 and built himself up. I'm quite proud of him as a son and as an admirer. But, the problem with my father is that he wants to write my future.

He is always telling me, or "reminding me" would be the suitable word, on how I was born with a golden spoon. Returning to the point, after a while living in that reality, I wanted to achieve something with my life. I wanted to build myself by myself without any help. I didn't want life to be as easy. I wanted Father to acknowledge me. Fortunately, when I was with a couple of peers, one day, I saw a boxing gym advertisement.

When I got home that day, I immediately opened my internet browser searching for boxing clips. I wanted to see what it was like to box. What is boxing? Should this be a sport? I remember the video I watched showcased Rocky Marciano. The other one I watched showcased Mohamad Ali. I was mesmerised! Two complete opposite styles but the exact same fierce personality. Rocky, standing like a man in front of his adversary and never backing down. Always stepping forward. Takes a beating like a man. On the other hand, Mohamed Ali lowering his guard and slipping through punches. Using his ring IQ to decide his counter's timing. Both were men. Men I dreamed of becoming one day. A man for my people. A man for my family. A man friends can lean on. A man of hope.

That day I decided after four minutes of watching Rocky Marciano and Mohamed Ali that I wanted to take up boxing. I went the next day to the advertised gym and the first words I told my coach before any greetings were "I'm not here to play. I'm only here to become a champion." My coach started laughing. I didn't change my facial expression. Subsequently, he realised I was serious. His laughter faded and his face altered to a serious one. "Get ready then. You have a long road ahead of you", is what he replied. I started training three times per week, then six times, and then eventually, I trained every day. Some days two times per day. Boxing consumed my life. I stopped going to my father's office. Obviously, he started getting ragingly upset. I didn't care. I wanted to feel like I was strong. I wanted to become a champion.

After training every day for half a year, I participated in my first nationals. It was my first-time cutting weight. It wasn't too hard for my body weight at the time was close to the weight I was competing at. I reckon I only had to cut 6.6 pounds (3kgs.). Regardless, in this competition, I grasped the feeling of what cutting weight is all about. I had to maintain my weight for six consecutive days. We would weigh in at 08:00 AM and compete by 11:00 AM. After the competition, we would eat our final meal and train at night to maintain our weight. I ended up finishing second place in the competition. It was heartbreaking. The tears that fell that day, I still feel them today. Anyhow, that was my first competition.

I ended up competing in a couple of more when I eventually stopped boxing for nearly six months due to my negligence when using a kitchen knife. Instead of slicing the apple, I sliced my thumb. In these six months, I only performed conditioning training to keep myself in shape. After these six months were done, I was in Romania at the time, and I got to train there for a while. I trained all three months of summer in a maddening way. I used to train two times per day usually and even three times per day, 30% of the time. My mind was consumed in becoming strong again. Two and a half months in and I fractured a rib. How did that happen, you ask? I wanted to compete in a boxing gala, but boxing wasn't the popular sport in the city I stayed in.

Thus, I ended up participating in a kick-boxing gala. During the match, I was confident in my upper skills, but unfortunately, I didn't calculate the distance warily, and he got me with his sidekick. At that moment, I couldn't breathe but guess what. I remembered what got me into boxing at that time. I saw Marciano's face taking a beating and never backing down or showing fear. I continued the match, and in the end I won by TKO.

After the gala, I realised the fracture was severe. I couldn't withstand deep breathes, could only sleep while being motionless and couldn't get out of bed. I literally felt like a disabled man. I felt weak. I didn't want to feel that way. Therefore, I took Diclofenac, a pain medication, and continued training. I would feel the pain after training.

I could use neither my left hook nor uppercut. Just slow clumsy jabs. Let me put it this way. Fancy throwing a mid-paced jab and just before you strike the mitts or heavy bag, someone would stab you in the ribs. That was the pain felt at the time. In days where I couldn't master the pain, I would swim for 1 hour. Upon returning to my country, I trained moderately every day for one month. I had no boxing training in this one month. By this time, it was I reason, 13-15th of October. I was at my high school when my sports teacher approached and informed me that the boxing competition was due on the 28th of this month. I was paralysed for a couple of minutes. My rib hadn't recovered yet. That meant I couldn't spar nor punch with my left arm. I was 13.2 pounds (6kgs) above my fighting weight which was 132.3 (60kgs). Without adding the fact that I had no boxing training for over a month. I didn't know what to do…

I'm just having a joke. Of course, I knew what I had to do. A fire lit in me. A new challenge. A new journey ahead of me. What's life without challenges? And thus, my esteemed readers, begins the journey.

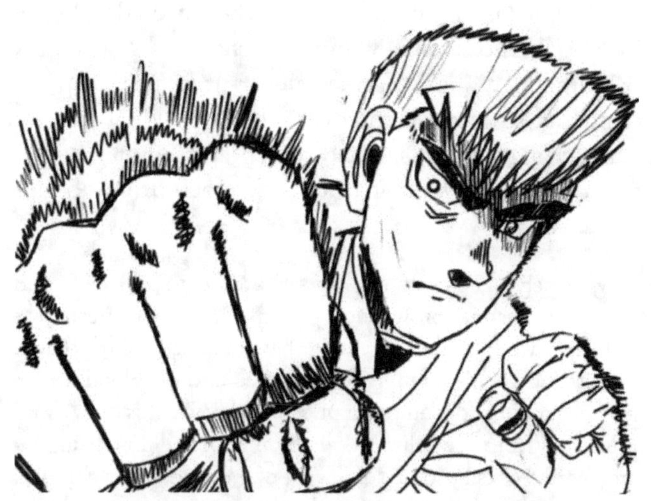

15-21ST OF OCTOBER

145.5LBS (66KGS)
13 DAYS LEFT

Initially, after hearing the competition's (qualifications for the nationals) date, I approached training more seriously and intensely. From the 15th till the 22nd, I would wake up at 05:00 AM and jog for about 3kms. Sometimes I would swim after running. Sometimes I would do body-weight training and conditioning. I would return home afterwards, take a shower, and go to school. I wouldn't eat breakfast. Just drink some water. Fasting helped me noticeably. Normally, I wouldn't go to school and sit at home, but fasting in addition to school would help me lose a pound or two. 7-8 hours of school would just pass by without me noticing the hunger. It helped keep my mind away from food and distracted. I would say it was a game changer for, if I would've slept instead of going to school, my body wouldn't burn those 500 or more calories at school.

After school, I customarily took a decent-sized plate and filled it with some brown rice, grilled chicken, and fresh vegetables. I would not eat anything that contained either sodium or salts for when sodium is administered into the blood, which may occur after consumption of salty food, water is drawn into the blood from the cells. Blood volume for the time being increases, the cells become somewhat dehydrated, and a complex hormonal response will eventually instinct the person to drink more fluid. Fluid intake offsets the temporary increase in blood sodium and reestablishes water balance. That is the brief scientific explanation on why I cut them from my meals.

I didn't measure my meals or anything at the time. I would just eat one chicken breast and half a cup of brown rice. With vegetables, I would eat a decent amount. Following the meal, I would take a nap, wake up, and leave for my boxing training. Training was intense. I used to train with an Olympic qualifier. Thus, his workouts were intense. Really intense. Some guys would puke in the middle of training. Before sleeping, I would eat one yoghurt. I customarily went to bed by midnight. That was my daily program for the first week. One meal a day. No sodas. No sweets. Just food that kept me going. Unfortunately, food was rather dry, I must say. Sometimes I altered the chicken with a salmon slice or a half can of tuna. Extreme hunger didn't hit in just yet at the time; only slight pain or hunger. But a type of hunger that I could endure, at least. In this week, I focused more on my technical boxing instead of weight cutting. I tried to have as much energy as I could during training as I knew that during the next week, my energy would plummet down a mountain. I may sound as if this week of training was easy, but I assure you it was no walk in the park.

Although I could endure the training, what made it harder was its repetitiveness. On the 5th day of the week, my body's soreness rose to its climax. I craved a day of rest but couldn't risk it. If I don't train, I get all frustrated and agitated. Training keeps me going.

In one of my notes dated 19th of October, I wrote, "My body is sore. Awfully sore. I cannot take it. I couldn't get out of bed this morning. My body hurt too much. I ended up taking an anti-inflammatory and a pre-workout supplement to help me endure the training. Upon reaching my 2nd km, it was all about the mind at that point. Every cell in my body was tenaciously calling for a halt."

This is no movie where I say I conquered myself and ran the entire distance. This was real life. I, unfortunately, and regrettably, winded down jogging to two and a half kilometres only. I couldn't take it. That's what it was. I was a bit down-hearted at the time, but I trapped those feelings away. I ended up skipping school that day for I figured my body needed rest and sleep. I hoped it would work.

I didn't eat much today. I assumed that my performance would downgrade and I wouldn't train that hard. Subsequently, I did some light stretching and went to my training. And as predicted, today's training went down the sink. I couldn't punch properly. My arms would start burning after 1 minute of shadowboxing. I Couldn't keep up during sparring.

I just felt like it was my first day of training. I skipped rope for half an hour after training was done to make myself feel better. And it worked. It motivated me to keep the days going at least.

The next two days where much better as the soreness faded a little. That was my first week. Now the real struggle came into play. On the morning of the 22nd, I weighed myself, and I came in at 138.8lbs (63kgs) which means I only lost 6 pounds in a whole week. It was heartbreaking, but I knew that this was how my body worked and I needed to cooperate with it. I had seven more pounds to go. I needed to be below 132.3 (60kgs) because if I came in even 0.1 pounds above the official weight, I would be disqualified. I needn't risk it. My goal was 131.1lbs (59.5kgs). For a couple of days, my diet altered slightly by drinking more water and reducing my portion sizes. By this point, hunger hit a homerun.

22ND OF OCTOBER

138.8LBS (63KGS)
6 DAYS LEFT

It was the first day of the week—a Monday. I did my morning run that day on the beach and swam for 2kms afterwards. Next Wednesday, I would prepare myself to swim 5kms. I am only accustomed to swimming on the beach. Sometimes I swim indoors but just when the weather is too unpleasant outside. Swimming helps me psychologically. I don't know the reason why, but while swimming, I feel stress-free. I forget my troubles and my life for these moments and fly through the sea's waves—carefree like the fish beside me.

I went to school just as usual that day. I got home, ate my small portion of food, and took a nap. I went to training with as little energy as my portion sizes. No power. I had no energy in me at all, but I kept going.

Today's training wasn't that satisfactory. It became demanding. When I got home today, I found my father waiting for me. He kept nagging me on how he wishes for me to hang my gloves and pursue a legitimate career. He didn't claim it, but I know he isn't satisfied with me. Everyone's expecting a lot from you. We ended up having a minor argument. I am distressed as a result. That's all I have to say.

23RD OF OCTOBER

138.6LBS (62.9KGS)
5 DAYS LEFT

O.2 pounds. I can't say I was satisfied at the time. Nothing special happened on this day, just the usual—the constant feeling of hunger. I just wanted to get on with the day at this point.

Throughout the week, I felt a constant strain on my lower back. I did not sit back and give it thought by then, but today during training, I began to feel tremendous pain from my right lower back to my ankle. I broke off halfway through my mitts workout. I couldn't take a step forward.

When I took a left step and started to twist my core to throw a straight right, the pain was unimaginable. I felt like I was paralysed at the time. I discussed the problem with my coach, and he suggested I take anti-inflammatory injections to keep me going through the training. If I took them constantly, would they lose their effect after a while? I needn't have asked this question for I needed the drug. The pain was too great. It was disappointing. Injury after injury. It's as if I was bad luck in the flesh. Today was a dire day.

24TH OF OCTOBER

138.8LBS (63KGS)
4 DAYS LEFT

Wednesday 24th. Feeling down-hearted. Weight doesn't come down as I want it to do. I woke up today feeling a bit better than yesterday. I don't feel the tear in my lower back as much. Today I was set to swim for 5kms. I went to the beach and ran for maybe 2kms as a warm-up and began to swim afterwards. It wasn't that hard but it wasn't easy either. It is just when you're happy doing something that time passes rapidly. It seems like happy moments last for seconds. I swam and kept on swimming. I kept my arms moving. Feeling the breeze of the sea. Watching the fish swim beside me, feeling the waves. It helped me consciously a great deal.

That day I ate nothing except for a can of tuna. No sides. Just tuna for the whole day. I drank as much water as I could for, I would dehydrate before the weigh-in and take out as much water as I could. I am in a worst-case scenario at this moment. I'm way more overweight than I expected. "It seems like I don't lose weight as I expected. I'll discuss this situation today with my coach during training", I thought to myself. I needed to take extra precautions so I wore my sauna suit beneath my outfit when I went into training. I loathe the sauna suit. But what can I do? It has to be done.

I couldn't keep up with the session today. Maybe it was because I am not used to the sauna suit yet. My heart rate went above the rooftop. The good part was that I looked like an avatar water bender. While walking, I was making water trails as if I was in *"Hansel and Gretel"*. I hope I took down 4 pounds, to say the least. I discussed my losing weight dilemma with my coach. He suggested taking "intense fat burner pills". I don't know what they are yet or if they have any side effects. I'll need to do some research until I decide whether I will take them or not. I will drink some water and dive into sleep. Another day is done. A couple more to go.

25TH OF OCTOBER

138.6LBS (62.9KGS)
3 DAYS LEFT

'm in despair. How come I don't lose weight. There is something wrong. Maybe. Just maybe it has to do with the water I drink after training. My weight before drinking and going to sleep was 137.5lbs (62.4kgs). Yes. It must be the water. Should I cut it out after training then? I think I'm in no position to debate the matter. I'll have to. Maybe take some sips to keep me from going mad.

I have woken up hungry. I'm quite hungry at this point. It is 06:10 AM. Came back from my morning jog with a weary look on my face. I made it through the run. My body, at this point, is telling me it isn't worth it.

That I should give up. It's a good thing I have a solid mind. I hope the hunger doesn't get worse for today I'll eat a salmon slice only." By that point, I was extremely hungry, but I wasn't hallucinating about food yet. I would watch food clips to keep me from thinking about food. I did my research about the fat burner pills that day, and I was sceptical on whether to take them or not. They had various kinds of side effects that varied from anxiety, increased heart rate, high blood pressure, insomnia, runny nose, sore throat, and headaches. I decided to wait for another day and instead see the results of my cutting water after training.

I came back from training. It was a discouraging session. I've got a black eye, and I've bled from my nose. Fortunately, my nose has not broken, yet. I was dreadfully sloppy. We wear no gear for protection during sparring. At least I've continued the session and kept sweating. I've weighed myself, and I came to 136.9lbs (62.1kgs). Will take some sips of water, and I am done for today. Nothing going through my mouth anymore. I am dreadfully hungry at the moment. Exceedingly starved. I'll have to fight through it by watching food clips. I stopped by the local supplement store on my way back home and bought the fat burner pills. I may need them. I hope not. I'm discouraged at the moment. I need to find the strength to keep going…

26TH OF OCTOBER

137.1LBS (62.2KGS)
2 DAYS LEFT

At this point, I feel better about my weight. As I suspected it was the water I drank after training. The only issue I have right now is dehydrating too early. I'll have to drink a decent amount of water before training. I told myself that I would wait until tomorrow to see if I would use the fat burner pills. By now, I walked through starvation's gate. No more hunger. Constant starvation. My mood changed. I couldn't speak to anyone. I was irritated all the time. I half a can of tuna all day. "I'll just need to hold on another day. Just another day and I can eat." This is the only thought going through my mind all day. I did my morning run. Afterwards, I ate my half a can of tuna and slept until training time. I wore the sauna suit again today. It was devastating. My heart rate increased to a high level, and it wouldn't decrease. I could feel the rapid heartbeats.

Due to the adverse weather conditions, I couldn't go to my boxing gym, so I went to a local gym instead. I ran for 5kms at an average pace of 8kms/hour. Afterwards, I did some shadow boxing for 10 rounds. Each round was 2 minutes long, and after each round, I would rest for 10 seconds. Let me be clear… I felt like my soul was being taken. It was extremely demanding. After I did my rounds, I just lay on the floor, placed a towel above my head, and sat there for half an hour until my heart rate started to decrease. I may have taken a quick nap by that point. I don't remember how time had passed so rapidly. All I remember is laying down and getting up. It was a hard training session. I couldn't even remove my outfit. I had no energy left in me. I may have stayed in the locker room an extra half an hour to just take my garments off. No strength at all. I weighed myself just now before I began writing these notes. I came at 134.4lbs (61kgs). I am happy with the results. I think if I fast for 24 hours before the weigh-in I would make it. Maybe I will rest tomorrow for I need some rest before the competition. I'll only drink some sips for my throat and mouth are dry. One more day to go.

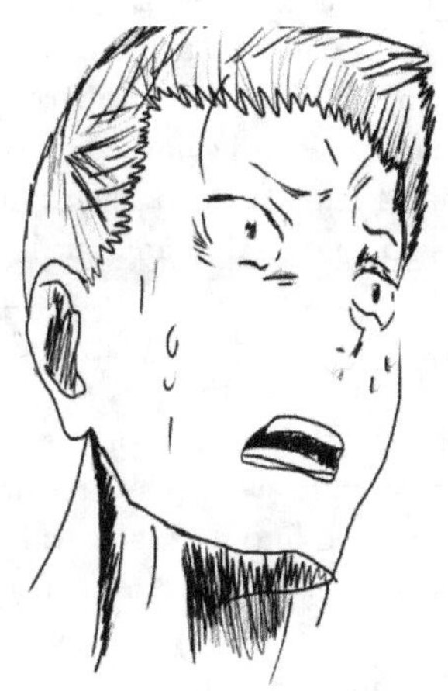

27TH OF OCTOBER
134.7LBS (61.1KGS)
24 HOURS LEFT

I don't know why I don't burn calories while sleeping. Is it because I don't sleep much? I've slept today for about 7 hours. More than enough in my opinion. Regardless, this day was one of the harshest. I woke up at 09:00 AM to eat my last meal and drink my last bit of water before I fast until the weigh in. I ate 1 boiled egg and drank my last sips of water. I weighed myself again and was up by 1 or 2 pounds. I decided afterwards to take 1 fat burner pill.

It was a huge mistake. After half an hour, the side effects began to show up. My heart rate increased, causing me to have anxiety and edginess. My nose became runny, and I developed a slight headache. I began having cold sweats. My hands began to shake, and I felt a feverish sensation. I wasn't ill. I don't know what was going on. After an hour I began to hallucinate. I would feel the cold sweat on my forehead. The most irksome side effect was the increased heart rate and anxiety.

I couldn't take this feeling anymore, so I put on some shorts and went to the beach to swim. The very first step into the cold sea relaxed me. I dived into the water without delay. Once I've dived into the water, my heart rate increased tremendously. I was happy. I just swam and swam. I was carefree. Just for a moment, I forgot about my life and felt more or less like a fish in the sea. I swam for about 45-minutes and bore the effect of swimming immediately. My heart rate decreased slightly, but my anxiety was half gone. I felt great. I still have 1 more pound to go. I hope it's gone by tomorrow. It's currently 10:30 PM. I'll go to sleep now for tomorrow I will ultimately get to eat.

28TH OF OCTOBER

131.6LBS (59.7KGS)

O4:30 AM… I can't sleep. Is it from the excitement? The fat burner pill? I just can't get to sleep. If I'm going to compete today, I'll need some rest, to say the least. I will try my luck once again…

05:00AM… FAIL…FAIL…FAIL… I CAN'T SLEEP. I need to sleep. I feel like I'm going mad. I contemplate about food. About how my performance is going to be like. I'm anxious. I don't know what to do at this point. My mouth is dry. I need to distract my mind with something. I need to, but I cannot concentrate on anything else except for food. I'll just need to hold on. Hold…on…

09:00 PM… Well, today didn't go as planned. I mean, it was really confusing. The system was ridiculous. It's as if the country's boxing federation doesn't give two shillings about us, the players. Let me elucidate… I had no sleep yesterday, so I stayed in bed until it was school time. I went to school and popped on the bus to get to the competition's location. We arrived there at about 09:00 AM. The sun was so bright that it could give us a tan even though we are already bronze. The place is all filled with dust and sand. It was in the open air. I thought I was in one of those cowboy movies. We literally had to wait another hour for the referees who would weigh us to arrive. It was bloody miserable. No tree to cast a shadow. The sun rays blasting straight in your face. Not to make it sound worse or anything, but we had to wait for them this whole hour while standing. Without mentioning the fact that some of the officials in attendance had chairs brought in for them to sit on while we stood in the bloody fire.

When the referees finally arrived, and we began to take our garments off to step on the scale, they suddenly started announcing that there had been a change in the weight divisions. "What the hell are they talking about?" was the thought that came to my mind. Are they for real? Do they mean to tell me that for those two weeks… two weeks of hell… they couldn't just make a call and inform us? Too hard of a task, right? Will drain their phones' credit.

Anyways, we encircled the referees to comprehend what exactly was going on. To make a long story short, my weight class division (132.3lbs (60kgs)) got disregarded. It was discouraging to see this kind of action from these people. We are supposed to be the future generation. The future of this country. But no. Apparently, they only cared about whether they're eating chicken or meat for dinner. I don't know why I'm ranting so much. I may be letting go of my frustration with these notes.

Nevertheless, after comprehending the situation, the only weight classes that I could've joined were the 125.6lbs (57kgs) weight class division and the 138.8lbs (63kgs) weight class division. That was one nightmare of a modification. At least, thanks to their MAJESTY, I got to choose which I could join. Who am I fooling? I had no options to decide from. Yes, they said I could choose which weight class I could join, but I was 131.6lbs (59.7kgs). I DON'T HAVE A FREE CHOICE. You might be thinking 'why don't I just go up in the weight class?' A simple answer to a simple question. I'll be competing tomorrow once more and by competing, I mean I'll have to weigh in… yet again. Thus, I'll be putting on the number of pounds left, with food and water. It's a bad idea… trust me. Fighters cut weight for when they rehydrate after weighing in, they would show up the day of the fight weighing 10 pounds or more. If I fight in the 138.8lbs (63kgs) weight division, I might find myself getting a nice ass whooping against adversaries greater in size. Anyhow, it's not like I had many choices to choose from.

They notified us about tomorrow's weigh-in location and time and set us to go. There were no matches that took part today. I'll get/have to play in the 138.8lbs (63kgs) weight class division. After all the hard work I put in, this happens. Anyway, at least I'll get to drink and eat more today. I did not rest. I went to training just as usual. I had much more energy in me. I could keep up easily with training. On the other hand, my friend, who got screwed over, just like myself over the weight division dilemma, had to lose 2-3 pounds. The weight class division he was supposed to compete in but got disregarded was the 141bs (64kgs) one.

He currently had to compete in my weight class division. He couldn't afford to choose the other weight division, which was 152.1bs (69kgs). It was too much of a jump. I advised him, "If you choose to add on those 13 pounds of weight, with food and water, somehow, over losing 2 or 3 pounds… you're screwed, man. Subsequently, he asked me for a fat burner pill to help him lose weight. That afternoon, during training, I found him wearing like 4 layers of garments. The guy couldn't even breathe. With that pill taking effect, he literally performed like an old geezer returning to the gym after a long period of rest. He clearly couldn't keep up with the training and had to lay on the floor for a good half an hour. I hope he loses those pounds. One weird day. I hope tomorrow goes well.

29TH OF OCTOBER

134.7LBS (61.1KGS)

Another day. One that was filled with emotion. The first quarter of the day was just infuriating. Basically, the location changed from yesterday's one. I went to the new location with two of my mates who were also competing. We arrived at a concrete basketball court. It was so small that I thought it was a kid's court instead, but it turned out it wasn't. Anyhow, behind one of the court's hoops was an underground room. It turned out that the cell sized room was the boxing gym. It wasn't that appealing, but we had to adapt. Essentially, there was no ring. Three green and outdated strings that were barely hooked to the wall formed the ring we were about to compete in. If a heavyweight suddenly decided to lean on these strings, the whole place would collapse. Nevertheless, this was where we would weigh in so all the players had to wait outside on the basketball court for the referees to arrive.

70 or more guys waited on the basketball court. We sat on concrete. An incalculable number of athletes sitting besides each other. It was distressing. To make matters worse, some

guys had to sit in the sun. Sweating beside each other, what were we waiting for? For the referees to arrive. I just don't believe how carefree they are. Some guys had to fast for 24 hours to make the weigh-in and needed to eat while those referees arrived 1 hour after the officially announced the time. It was infuriating. Anyhow… anyhow… after 1 hour of just waiting there, they finally arrived. We took off our garments and waited for our names to be called. After standing in the cold breeze for about 5 minutes, my name was finally called. I went in and came in at 134.7024lbs (61.1kgs). Both of my mates departed to buy us some food for we would supposedly compete after 3 hours. But yet again I'm mesmerised by this system. After they departed to buy the food, a referee came out of the underground room and announced several names. The names that were not announced were qualified for nationals. After asking around, I learned that in every weight class division, there were 4 spots available. If more than 5 guys weighed in at the same weight class division, they would have to compete against each other. In the end, my mate and I were off, we got qualified. My other mate, on the other hand, had to compete to qualify.

The other hindrance was that we basically just weighed in 10 minutes ago and a referee informed us that the announced players would compete immediately. Consequently, the dehydrated guys who were announced and didn't get a chance to rehydrate got screwed. And… my mate was one of them (Let's call him N). I called him immediately informing him about the news before he had anything and stuffed his belly. When he got back, I told him to get his blue outfit out and get outfitted. My other mate informed me, while N got outfitted, that from nervousness, N pulled his genitals out beside a tree in the middle of the walkway and decided to do his bathroom work there. He was extremely nervous. I don't blame him. It was his first competition. Not mentioning the fact that he was about to compete against a national champion. Once I informed him about this fact, he took his hand wraps off and said "I'm not playing… I'm not competing" and started packing his bag to leave. I shook his head and told him "It's ok. Just do your best" he regained his composure so I told him to do some muscle stretches. I literally turned around for a second, and when I looked back at him again, I suddenly found him doing knee-ups and jumping jacks. "WHAT IN THE WORLD ARE YOU DOING?"

"I don't know. I don't know." The guy was completely terrified. I threw some water on his face and told him to relax. Seemingly, we were competing with our own gloves, so I gave him his gloves and told him to do his best. I wasn't allowed to be his second. But apparently, upon my return to the basketball court, the crowd of guys just rushed through the boxing room, and the room was completely filled with people. There were a couple of windows, and I was able to get a glimpse of what was going on.

The referee called both players in the middle of the ring to salute each other and afterwards each player would return to their corner to wait for the bell. Apparently, N did not know that. Once N saluted his opponent, he punched him with a straight right jab. I lost my head. I was laughing hysterically. It was hilarious. I heard one of the judges yelling at him for his actions. The best part about it is that N had the face that expressed exactly what was going on in his head: "What did I do wrong?" It was too embarrassing. I couldn't watch the match. Unfortunately, N lost the match by TKO. Or was it? I watched the match since my mate filmed it. It seems that N was being counted upon. N was so outraged he was being counted against that he totally forgot to look at the referee and raise his guard up. Instead, he kept looking at his opponent with an outraged face. It was one hell of a day. Good thing he was not down-hearted after the game. At least he got his experience.

"We were informed about the location and the date of the Nationals competition, and we left. My mate and I stopped by a burger site and ate 6 pounds worth of food. I am home right now. The competition date is due to the 17th of October. I'll rest for a couple of days, and I'll be back for training and dieting but for now… I'll just rest my head off."

30TH OF OCTOBER
130LBS (59KGS)

I did not wake up for the morning run. I chose to rest my muscles as much as I could. I was eating miserably at that point. Sugars, sodas, and fried food. You name it. It was a mistake on my part. Anyhow, I went to my boxing training just as usual. We were doing some shadow boxing when I realised I might have torn my chest-shoulder area. I didn't know which part exactly for it expanded but every time I threw a hook or an uppercut, I would suffer immense pain coming from my left arm. All these injuries. I didn't know what to do anymore. I thought, perhaps, it was a onetime suffering so I shook it off that night and went to sleep without being…. anxious.

31TH OF OCTOBER

134.4LBS (61KGS)
19 DAY LEFT

I was willing to rest on this day for I thought that I over trained myself. My diet was still miserable. Eating junk food and all this bad stuff that you do not need. I got a phone call from a referee. He asked me if I was the right guy he's talking to, I approved. He mentioned that there had been a problem with the signing of names. I asked him what did he mean exactly, and he answered, "Look, your name wasn't written in the 138.8lbs (63kgs) weight class division. There has been a mistake. I called to inform you that you will have to go down to the 125.6lbs (57kgs) weight class division for there is a spot available. I'm sorry for the trouble we're causing you. What's the course of action you're going to take? I need to know in a couple of minutes."

What an organised federation. A brilliant federation and system. Distress shows up every couple of days. Nevertheless, I told him that I would call him immediately for I needed time to reflect on the matter. To be candid, I desired that drop. I was pleased with dropping to that division for it was my natural division that I competed at. I called my coach to inform him about the state of affairs, and I was surprised to know that the referee called him after our call. The surprising part was that my coach had already given him an answer which was that I would drop to the division mentioned. "Things are getting serious now" was my thought at the time. I was supposed to rest for the day, but after hearing this kind of news, I got excited. My heart rate increased. A fire was lit inside of me. I felt alive once again. Obviously, I couldn't train thoroughly for I kept thinking about my chest-shoulder tear. Train, train, and train was my train of thought. I didn't care much for the tear at the time

1ST AND 2ND OF NOVEMBER

143.3LBS (65KGS)
17 DAYS LEFT

On these 2-3 days, I trained moderately. My body needed some rest; therefore, I didn't train intensely. My diet, however, was chaotic. I couldn't maintain myself. I ate everything that was in my way. It was a grave mistake. I did not wish to step on the scale. I was too anxious about the number that was going to show up. Nonetheless, nothing special occurred on these dates. It was rather like a small holiday. "I will need to step up the game soon. Maybe tomorrow will officially be day one of training."

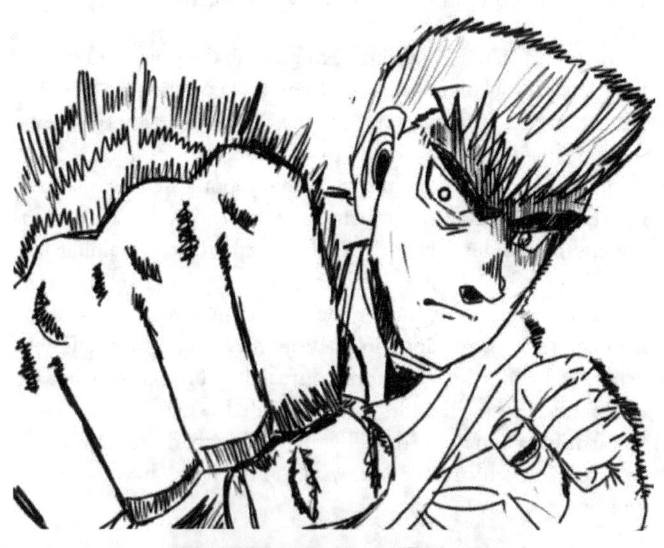

3RD OF NOVEMBER

147.7LBS (67 KGS)
14 DAYS LEFT

I woke up today and was determined to jog on the beach swim afterwards for a while. I ran for about 45 minutes at mid-pace. I did some stretches afterwards and hopped into the sea. Upon starting to swim, I realised my injury was severe. I couldn't swim. Couldn't get my left arm to peddle. What do you think my rational course of action was? I commenced swimming. I did not stop. I fought through the pain. I don't know why I did that. I wanted to keep rotating my arms. Perhaps I was releasing out my irritations and distress into the water. Perhaps so…

Anyhow, I lasted for about 20 minutes in the water before the pain was excruciating. I realised I couldn't continue like this, so I called for an appointment with my doctor. The appointment was on the same day, so after I was done with training, I went to the appointment. The result of this appointment was somehow disappointing. He confirmed my suspicions of having torn my chest-shoulder muscle. He advised me to stop training for a week, prescribed some medicine, and suggested an injection that would help me conquer the pain if needed. After calling my coach and informing him, he told me "forget him… Don't listen to doctors." I was more confused. Didn't know what to do. Should I rest? Should I train? I decided to take it easy on my left arm for a couple of days. I would only run, do some fitness, work on some footwork, and work on the heavy bag and mitts with my right arm.

Starting from today, I will begin my diet. No junk food, no sugars, no to anything that makes you fat. I'm back to my normal weight, even fatter. 147.7lbs (67 kgs) therefore I'm about to lose 24.2 (11 kgs) pounds in the next 2 weeks. That's quite a number of pounds. I perceive that 2-3 pounds is mainly food weight inside my belly. But the same amount of work would be done either way. For the next couple of days, I would only eat one meal per day and see how my progress would go. Today I ate a bowl of salad with unseasoned grilled chicken. I don't season my food. The chicken wasn't that dry for the salad moistened it. I went to my boxing training as usual today, and it was intense. I had to, or perhaps I will have to, level up my workouts to make up for my left arm. It's a fact. I will have to work extra hard. I can't shadowbox properly, can't use the heavy bag nor mitts the usual way, and most importantly, I can't work on my combinations. I'm only anxious for what if my arm does not heal? I'll be screwed. Even so, I will have to compete. 1st day done… 13 more to go.

FROM 4TH TILL 8TH OF NOVEMBER

142.2 (64.5KGS)
13 DAYS LEFT

These were nightmare days. Although I still enjoyed them. They were like the silence before the storm or the apocalypse. I enjoyed training at that point, even though it was extremely hard. I had the energy to finish my training, but during the last day or two, I felt my energy plummeting. "My weight isn't going as calculated. I will have to turn to desperate measures and use the fat burner pills. My trainer advised me to reach my desired weight before the weigh-in date with 2-3 days. I will have to use them."

I Did not feel my injury much. I restrained from using my left arm as much as possible. The morning training session, school, eat, nap, boxing session, and sleep - that was my customary program. Hope all goes well in these couple of days for I can feel a slight rush of fever. I hope I'm wrong.

FROM 4TH TILL 8TH OF NOVEMBER

9TH & 10TH OF NOVEMBER

140LBS (63.5 KGS)
8 DAYS LEFT

These days were hell for me. I have a fever, and even though I have it, I still need to go and train. I went yesterday to my boxing session, and the coach advised me to, "Go to your local gym, wear your sauna suit, run for a couple of kms, skip for half an hour, and finally enter the sauna for 15 minutes. You will feel better." During today's training session, he asked if I was feeling better. "Feeling better", he said? The whole time throughout the training program he has given me was as if I'm inside an oven. My heart rate was at its highest point. I couldn't breathe. My muscles were just crying for help. I came home today devastated. Can't even lift an arm. I was on the point of tearing. I had a runny nose through those two days. To make matters worse, that damned pill was taking its effect. I was anxious every minute of the day. The hunger came

in finally. Not that I was waiting for it. The starvation did
not hit me yet. My weight did not make that drastic of a
change. I'll wait to see tomorrow's morning weigh-in and
will decide whether I alter my diet or not.

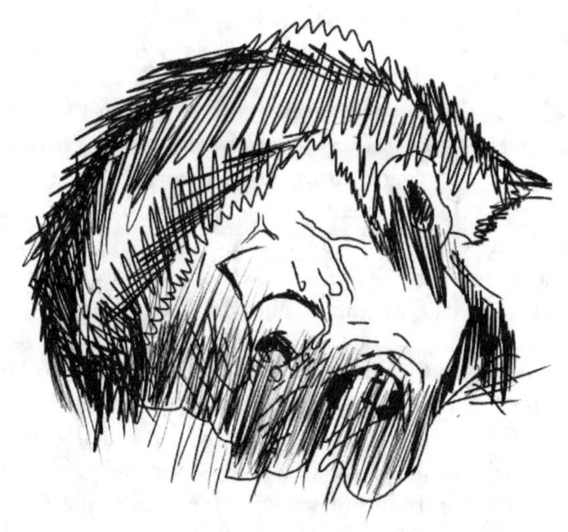

11TH OF NOVEMBER
139.4 (63.25 KGS)
6 DAYS LEFT

'm living in hell. I can't take it anymore. I am thinking of dropping the whole matter." Those were my words at 04:10 AM. Basically, my fever was as bad as it could get, the number on the scale would not go down, my left arm did not heal yet, and my mental condition was beginning to grow worse. I did not sleep the day before for I was hallucinating and pondering about food all the time.

I was watching food clips 24/7. I couldn't do anything else to waste my time. I tried watching movies, playing video games and reading. Nil effects. I still kept constantly pondering about food. I became short-tempered. I constantly thought of how I had one week left to endure. I was beginning to doubt if I would make it. It was too much. I went to the pharmacy to ask for some medicine for my fever. I required some medicine at this point. I was quite ill. My diet altered to either 1 chicken breast, 1 slice of salmon, or half a can of tuna per day. I will wait and see the results of this diet for a day or two and upon then, I will decide whether to alter my diet or not.

My mind was collapsing but I needed to train. I couldn't sit at home. I wore my sauna suit and went to training. I began to use my left arm during that day of training. It didn't go as I've anticipated. I still had the injury. My coach suggested to take Betamethasone. I did not know what it was at the time, so I told him that I will see. I arrived home done; tired of this whole competition.

I went to bed, but I couldn't sleep. I had hallucinations about food stores, chocolates, and all the good stuff. I couldn't take it. I went to the fridge, opened it, and kept staring and gazing at the food for some minutes. I just kept standing there, contemplating on my life. On whether it was worth it or not. My mind was hunting me. Food was hunting me. My mind was collapsing. I was about to just let it all out. I took a rice cake in my hand and was about to place it in my mouth, but I held it motionless within my mouth's reach. I was in despair. I gave in and chewed that damn thing, but I did not swallow it. I spit it straight into the trash. Afterwards, I bent down on my knees and began to whimper. "Why am I doing this to myself. Why!?"

I got back up and tried to go to bed. I couldn't. I had insomnia. I couldn't sleep. I was stuck in time, motionless in my bed. All alone. At about 3:00 AM in the morning, I got up and went to the living room. From the living room's balcony in my apartment, you can view the sea. And that was my course of action. Standing, staring at the sea.

I did not keep track of the time, but for a moment I felt sound again. I've forgotten that I'm starving, forgotten about my injuries, and forgotten about the expectations from me. I was a fish for a moment. I wished I could be able to swim in the sea but unfortunately, couldn't. The weather and my fever… Afterwards I came back to reality. I was starving once more. I had to watch some food clips to forget about starvation. I don't know how it worked, but it helped. While watching, I laid on the couch and tried to sleep. My eyes were aching, my nose was runny, and my mind was in despair. "I'm living in hell. I can't take it anymore. I am thinking of dropping the whole matter." And after noting this sentence, I stayed awake the whole night. Hallucinating from time to time about reality. Dreary…

12TH OF NOVEMBER
135.5LBS (61.5KGS)
5 DAYS LEFT

This may be a night for you, but it surely wasn't for me. I was wide awake through the whole night. I went to school for I had an exam. I felt miserable. The weather was cold. My mates were having a laugh, while I was spaced out the whole time. Halfway through the exam, my brain just stopped processing things. My heart rate was raised for I took a fat burner pill in the morning. I felt sick to my stomach. I wanted to eat more than anything. Now starvation became grave. I didn't fancy the food I craved for anymore. I sought after anything edible, even the food I detested. I, ironically, evolved to my predecessor's survival instinct. I wanted any edible food. At that right moment, I still remember it perfectly, I thought to myself, "Why don't I just give up. Maybe I'll just go home and eat. Why am I doing this? No one knows the pain I'm going through anyways. Just look at them. All carefree. All of them…" I was on the verge of letting it all go…

I asked my chemistry teacher about Betamethasone, and it was one hell of an insight to know about the drug. My teacher was taken aback with a bewildered face. When I asked her why this reaction, she replied, "Don't you know? Betamethasone has cortisone, which are basically steroids. Isn't it illegal in sports?" I then put her into the picture and disclosed my tear injury. I also told her that my coach was the one suggesting them for pain-relief "but it stays in the blood for six whole months. Afterwards it weakens your bones. Other side effects include acne, gaining weight, and stretch marks. I wouldn't recommend it", and by that, we concluded our conversation. What an insight. I don't think I will take the risk. Too risky. I will have to fight through the pain, or more precisely said, fight with the pain."

When I got home that day, I ate my slice of salmon and went to sleep. I didn't want to think about food. I wanted to distract myself as much as possible. I ended up going to training with my flu. The process became unenjoyable. No more fun. I had to fight through the day without cracking up. The worst part of the day is at night. Lonely in my thoughts. No one besides you but the voice inside your head. If that voice was in flesh and blood, I would've murdered it. I was going crazy. Voices in my head kept telling me to give up and eat. To open the fridge and eat it up. I would stay awake for 5 hours in bed with my own thoughts. Hallucinating. Cracking up. On the verge of letting it all go. All go. "I'm still hanging in there though. Still hanging."

13TH OF NOVEMBER

133.3LBS (60.5KGS)
4 DAYS LEFT

My flu doesn't appear to be as grave as yesterday. I still have a fever though. I had a good sleep last night. Even though I went to sleep at dawn. I stood on the scales. Viewing the number, I realised the trouble I'm in. Weight was not going down. What else could I do? To what extent would I reduce my food portion sizes. But what can I do? It had to be done. Only 1 boiled egg per day from now on. I drank as much water as I could today for by tomorrow, I would reduce my water intake. As you have been accustomed to by now, I was in despair 24/7. I had to try to distract myself through the day. I couldn't watch boxing clips to study them. It would increase my heart rate with excitement and rush the blood in me. I didn't need that right now. I watched food clips. The only thing I could keep on watching.

Today's training was dreadful. My nose bled again. I sparred with an amateur who thought boxing was the same as brawling.

I didn't know his style at first, but when we began, I perceived him rushing with wild punches and headbutts. I didn't have the energy to fight, but then after bleeding and noticing his face with a smirk on it, I snapped. If he wanted a brawl, I would give him a war. I knocked him out. Showed him he's an amateur after all. My nose kept bleeding though. I was disappointed, but now my energy was drained. I hadn't the energy to take notes anymore.

The best thing that happened on that day was immediately after writing these notes, I slept. I was able to sleep. I was extremely satisfied on the day afterwards. At least it gave me a slight relieve in this pile of haystack. A good night's sleep…

14TH OF NOVEMBER

131.6LBS (59.7KGS)
3 DAYS LEFT

It is 2:00 AM in the morning of the 15th. I can't sleep. In the next couple of days, it would be as hard as surviving in the desert searching for water. I am as desperate at the moment. I need water. I need food. I have a cold sweat. I keep hallucinating things. I can't think properly. I don't know what to do anymore. I'm on the verge of giving up. I blackout every time I stand up. My mind just shuts off for a couple of seconds. I see darkness. My eyes blackout completely. My head becomes extremely heavy and begins to swirl. I keep holding on and standing... I don't know how much I can take it any longer. I don't know. Why? WHY?!

The blackout thing was causing me major difficulties. While standing up, I would black out completely. Almost every time I was on the verge of falling. Those couple of days were like hell for me. I remember that day, for when I was at school the sport's teacher gave my mate and me the money for our competition. Essentially, money for accommodation, food, and transport. They gave us what turns around to be $20 for each of us. It was money for 2 days. It was nothing. We obviously had to travel on our own expenses. They told us the competition's location and wer departed on our journey. I wouldn't wish this experience for my nemesis. I can't recall very much from the 14th till the weigh-in day, except for minor episodes. I seem to have forgotten almost everything. All I can give you are the notes I have written at the time…

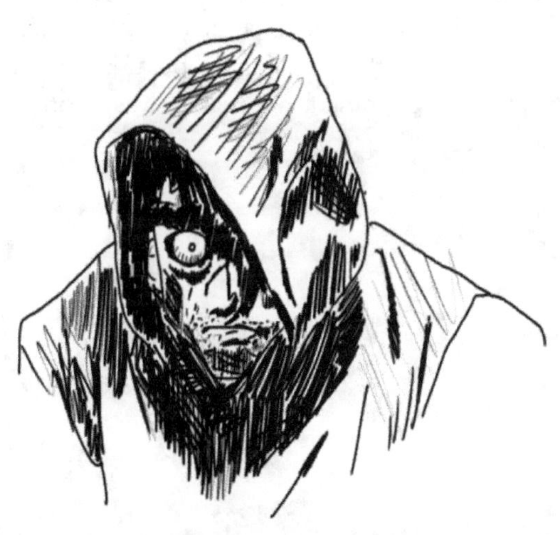

15TH OF NOVEMBER

130.5LBS (59.2KGS)
2 DAYS LEFT

Why am I doing this? I can't keep it up. I've been in this state for a month now. My head. My throat. I need water. I don't need food anymore. I just require water. I only drink sips. I need more. MORE. I whimpered during training. I couldn't stand up, but I kept moving. I couldn't hold my guard, but I kept punching. When training was finally over, I went to my knees, placed my head on the floor, and whimpered. I kept asking myself for a reason on why I don't just give up. Then I remembered, I wanted to know the meaning of being strong. To be a MAN. A hero for myself. My reason was strong enough for me to keep going forward.

—

When I got home and weighed myself, my weight was the same. Only a pound lost throughout the day. I despaired. I wore my shoes and went for a run. I was too anxious to stay at home, so I ran. I'm in despair. I want water. My mouth is dry. The sips don't work anymore. Tomorrow. Tomorrow, I will depart to the location where the competition is taking place. I will need to make it through this last night. I have to. Just a few hours left and I can drink…

I vaguely remember that day, but I remember some of the instances when I was out running. I remember I kept saying to myself while running, "RUN. RUN. RUN. KEEP RUN-NING. KEEP HOLDING ON. KEEP HOLDING ON". It was truthfully one of the toughest, if not the most demanding times of my life. My mouth was extremely dry. I only drank sips of water for my weight. It was dreadful. I was in a dreary state. I wanted to get on with the day. I only had a couple of hours left. I only needed to get through the night…

16TH OF NOVEMBER

128.9LBS (58.5KGS)
24 HOURS LEFT

I only slept for about 2 hours today. When I woke up, I checked the scale immediately. I was furious. I needed to lose a couple more pounds. My hell wasn't ending. I wore my sauna suit and took drastic measures. I had a built-in sauna at home; therefore, I made use of it. Here's how it went:

- I entered the sauna for 15 minutes.

- I went out and skipped rope for 10 minutes.

- I went back to the sauna for 10 more minutes.

- Finally, I went out and skipped rope for 5 minutes.

The trouble was that after finishing, I remembered that I hadn't drunk nor eaten. By that, I mean neither sipped some water or had a bite of a boiled egg. The pressure from my weight made me forget about my thirst. But lastly and after a long road, I got down to my weight, technically. I'm still 126.1lbs (57.2kgs), but I will lose those 2-3 pounds before my weigh in. No more running, no more skipping, and no more training. It's a patience game presently. All I have to do is wait.

I'm set to leave my city at 5:00 PM. It is currently 1:00 PM. I will relax till departure time…

1:00 AM. It was one of the most infuriating/degrading travels I've ever had. We departed and travelled in my car. I had a driving license, but I chose not to drive for it would've been too risky. I asked my uncle to drive us instead. It was a 4-hour drive, but it felt like 1-hour instead. There was a hotel near the competition's site, and therefore we were supposed to stay there until the end of the competition. It did not work out that way.

There were no rooms available. Yes… Not a single one. We did not know what to do. The other trouble we faced was that we were not familiar with the city we were in. I asked my uncle to drive us to near hotels that were suggested on my phone's maps. We ended up visiting 5 total hotels. NO HOTEL HAD AVAILABLE ROOMS! You would say, "Well it is your fault. Who asked you to travel without booking a room?" You're partly right but, in my defence, the location was confirmed on the 14th. I had no time to book. In all events, we ended up in a hotel that was a little expensive. Making the matters worse, it was a 1-hour drive from the competition building. Good thing I asked for to leave the car…

My uncle left us. We are in our rooms at the moment. the weigh in is tomorrow at 3:00 PM. These judges and referees seem to make matters easy for themselves. It was supposed to be at 08:00 AM in the morning, but they changed it. It seems they are heavy sleepers. This boxing federation is corrupt. They don't care about the guys who sweat and starve themselves for the weigh in. I even saw one of the judges in the hotel that was near the competition's building. I presume all of them are staying there. They get to rest as much as they want while we will have to wake up an hour and a half before the weigh in to just make it in time…

I did not feel my starvation as much today. The excitement from the journey and having a mate amongst my side helped. Although he farted while sleeping and I had to sleep with the bed covers over my head, it's still a decent thing to have him by my side. Tomorrow's the weigh-in. Hope all goes well…

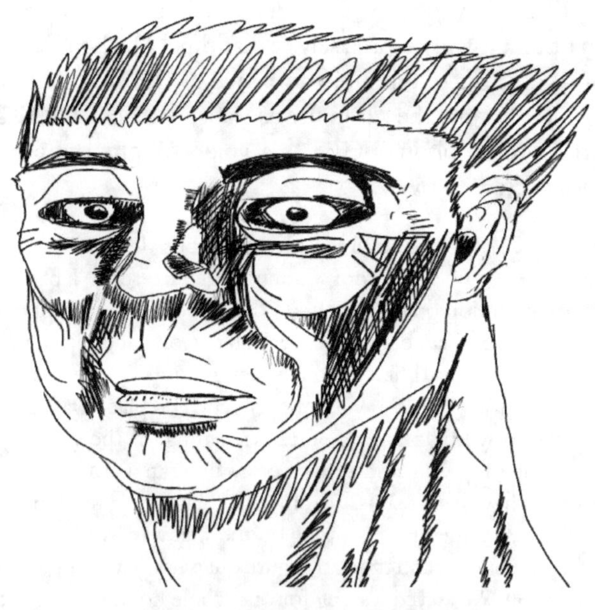

17TH OF NOVEMBER

WEIGHT???

12:30 PM. One of the best night's sleep I've ever had. I nearly slept for twelve hours. Even though I woke up tired and had no energy in me, I felt relaxed. I don't know my weight at the moment, but I'm confident that I have made it. We don't have a scale in our room. The hotel's gym scales do not work. Luck isn't on our side. We decided to leave the hotel by 2:00 PM. Weigh-in is at 3:00 PM. Knowing how the federation and referees are, I don't think it will be precisely at that time. Maybe by 4:00 PM. We will take one hour to arrive to our destination. My uncle left me the car to use as transportation. I'll have to rely on the phone's GPS as a guide. I hope the GPS doesn't screw us over.

It was a long road until we arrived at our destination. My heart rate was over the roof during the entire road. I had to keep my attention on the road and GPS while my mate slept beside me. I don't blame him. We were quite worn out. Upon our arrival, we perceived like 200 guys waiting outside the boxing building. It was 3:10 PM when we arrived. The place was filled with this crowd of people. Some were sitting on the walkway, some beside the wall, and some were waiting in a coffee shop. Basically, they were teams. We, my mate and I, were alone… Regardless, I remember us sitting on the walkway. We kept observing the players and trying to figure out who may compete in our division. We stayed waiting for one whole hour. One whole hour. These referees have no sense of respect. I swear. Some of us were literally fasting for 30+ hours. My mouth was so dry that I couldn't even talk. My lips were dehydrated to the point at which I couldn't move them or else I would feel pain. No sense of respect at all!

When they finally arrived, crowds began making their way through the gate. It felt like Black Friday. Before the official weigh-in, we had to do the experimental weigh-in to see if we need to lose a pound or two. If you are above your stated weight with even 0.1lbs (0.05kgs), you are disqualified immediately. Consequently, 200 guys had to stand in a line to weigh in. You had to push your way through the line so that you could get a chance to weigh in or else these guys would push you or stand in front of you. It was miserable. Chaotic. Eventually, we, my mate and I, weighed in and we came under our official weight with a couple of pounds. The referees then announced that the official weigh-in was in half an hour as some guys came in above their official weigh.

Thus, the referees had to give them a reasonable amount of time for them to be able to lose these extra pounds. My mate and I got out of the building and waited outside for it was chaotic inside. A bunch of guys got in the ring and started to jump, move around, and take God damn pictures. It's as if they haven't seen a ring before. Although it was the best ring in the country, for it was the one where the Olympic national team trained in, but still. While waiting outside, we perceived guys skipping rope, jogging, shadow boxing, and doing some fitness. I mean, I don't want to hate, but they deserve this. I worked hard to go down to my weight; they didn't work as hard. Re-gardless, my friend couldn't hold on to his fast so he bought a bag of popcorn and ate it. I couldn't afford to do that. After half an hour, we got back inside, took off our garments, and stood in the line for the official weigh-in.

While standing in line with my underwear, I perceived that one of the referees was looking towards me in a queer way. When we made eye contact, he suddenly cried, "go and shave your beard or else I won't allow you to weigh." GOOD LORD! I didn't even have a beard. It was a five-o'clock shadow beard. I was in awe. I tried to make my way through to the scale, but he made it impossible for me. Consequently, I ran through the hall with my underwear covering me, and then I find the security guy crying that I wasn't allowed to walk through the hall with my underwear. I went back to the gym, wore some shorts and my mate's shirt and went to the bathroom.

A bunch of other guys were doing what I was about to do. The trouble was, I didn't have a razor with me. I found one that wasn't in use besides the sink. Obviously, some other guy used it, but I hadn't the time to think twice. I took it and shaved my face like never before. I had the babyface shave. Afterwards, I weighed in, and I was finally done. There's an important fact I need to state, though. We were informed that the weigh-in was for only one day. That means, instead of weighing in every day like the usual, we would weigh in only once, which we did a couple of minutes ago. Which also means that I'm done with the diet and all that crap.

After the weigh-in, I drank a bottle of water with some energy drink and ate popcorn. The referees then informed us that we would need to wait until the judges schedule the matches. We thought it would take half an hour or so. Boy where we wrong. BOY WHERE WE WRONG. It was 17:00 PM when we first went outside to wait. We sat in the freezing cold till 8:00 PM, and they still had not finished. We haven't eaten ANYTHING yet. We had to wait to confirm that the weigh-in was for only a day.

During this waiting interval, we met a guy that my mate and I became friends with. We sat together outside, waiting for their majesty to relieve us from this situation so we can leave. Keep in mind, we were still a one-hour drive away from our hotel without forgetting the fact that I am the one who is going to drive there while starving. During the interval, we were literally shocked. We then observed the judges, by maybe 6:30 PM having a dinner break. It was really infuriating to perceive such actions. At least we got to see the Olympic boxing team train. That kept us distracted while waiting. By 8:15 PM we had it confirmed from a coach, whom we saw talking to the judges, that the weigh-in is for only one day.

The only remaining issue is the match schedule. I wasn't going to wait anymore. I gave our friend whom we met my number and asked him to call and inform us about it. We greeted him and left. We decided to stop by a burger place to celebrate making the weigh-in and eat as much as possible. As much as we were starving, we were relieved. No more dieting. We ordered two burgers for each of us. The hardest part was waiting for the order to arrive. When it ultimately came, halfway through the second burger, I got a phone call. "Yes?"

"Yeah, it's me M-… I called to inform you that weigh-in will not be for a day… weigh in shall take place everyday… your division is competing tomorrow by the way. Your mate will not be. He still needs to weigh in though…"

I didn't even reply to him afterwards. I just stared at my phone and my mate. "What is happening right now. Are these bunch of referees for real? Weigh-in every day?" These questions were swerving through my head. I was paralysed for a couple of minutes. Just staring vaguely. My mind shut off. "What should we do now?" Was the question we asked ourselves. We just ate 5 pounds worth of food. "What's the best strategy to take?" We obviously left the remaining food uneaten. We stopped by a local supermarket to buy some stuff and went to our hotel. During the drive back to the hotel, there was solely stillness. No music. No radio. Merely silence. We felt like… how should I say it… nothing. We felt nothing. We were in vagueness. In a vague mental state. We didn't know why this was happening to us. What were we even trying for…? All this pain and misfortune. Regardless of all this and after all the hard work we put into this, we weren't going to back down now.

If I remember correctly, we stepped inside our room at around 10:30 PM. My mate got an idea which was to puke all the food he had eaten. Immediately after stepping inside the room, he took the scale which we bought and weighed himself. He came in above his official weight by 3 pounds. He afterwards went to the bathroom to start puking. I heard his agony while trying to puke, and I couldn't hold my laughter even though we were in a distressed state. He also began laughing while puking when he heard my laughter. The noise his puking made sounded like water pouring into the toilet. After 5 minutes he came out of the bathroom and stepped onto the scale.

I was in disbelief. HE ACTUALLY PUKED 4 POUNDS! I wasn't going to try this method, but after seeing his results, I had nothing to lose but pounds so I gave it a try. Before I puked, I weighed myself, and I came 4 pounds above my official weight. I asked my mate how he has done it, and he elucidated with illustrations: Take two of your fingers and shove them inside your mouth while keeping them inside. I went into the bathroom, bent down, shoved my fingers inside, and tried to puke.

I was in agony. Nothing came out. NOTHING. At one point, I did not even know whether I was laughing or crying. What in the name of GOD was I doing? Why did I have to go through all this agony? At another point, I took a pen and shoved it inside instead of my fingers. Nothing. My Testicles began to hurt. I couldn't puke. After a quarter of an hour of futile trying, I finally gave up on this method.

The other methods that I was about to try were painful. Quite painful. Plenty of fighters have died while performing it. But after all, it had to be done. I took some trash bags, poked some holes in them, and wore the bloody things. Afterwards, I filled the bathtub with hot water and salt. Plenty of salt. While waiting for the bathtub to fill, I skipped rope for about 15 minutes to work out some sweat. After finishing with the rope, I stepped inside the bathtub. It was bloody hot. I felt like my skin was melting down. Perhaps it was the effect of the salt. Regardless, the plan was the following:

- Stay in the bathtub for 15 minutes.

- Get out, wrap myself up in towels, and wait for 10 minutes.

- Get back inside the bathtub and stay for another 10 minutes.

That was the presumed plan. And as you're already accustomed to, my plans don't go as anticipated. I couldn't perform it completely. I only stayed in the bathtub for 10 minutes and wrapped in towels for 5 minutes. It was too much agony. I hoped it did the job, though. It didn't… I only lost 2 pounds. I did not know if those 2 pounds left would go down in my sleep.

I needn't risk it. I took laxatives. By that point, I couldn't talk anymore. I nearly collapsed while coming out of the bathroom. The weigh-in was set to be at 9:00 AM the next day. We had to be awake by 7:30 AM. I only wrote one sentence in my notes that day "still hanging in there…"

18TH OF NOVEMBER

WEIGH-IN DAY

I woke up at about 06:00 AM with my stomach aching. I realised it was the work of the laxatives. I jumped out of bed and went to the bathroom. After relieving my bowels, I decided to check my weight. I did it. I weighed in under my official weight with 0.5lbs (0.2kgs). I went back to sleep afterwards with a relieved mind.

We woke up at about 7:30 AM. I prepared my bag, placing my gloves, hand wraps, competition's outfit, mouth guard, Vaseline, a power drink, and a chocolate bar inside.

We arrived at our destination at around 09:00 AM. While entering the building, we noticed that a referee was standing beside the weighing in room, and saying that the weigh-in will end soon. I immediately took off my garments and entered the room. I stood beside the scale waiting for the referee to ask me to stand on the scale. Once he gave me approval, I stepped on it. I at once tried to look at my weight, but the referee cried asking me to raise my head and look straight. I had shivers run through me. Even though a couple of seconds passed, it felt like hours till he finally asked me to step down. He informed me that I had 3 hours until the competition, and I subsequently walked outside. It was a relief.

After walking outside the building, I realised I had another setback which was that I had to wait 3 hours until the competition time. What was the point of going back to the hotel if the amount of time till we get there is one hour? We had to wait near the place. We found a couple of chairs by the side of the building and sat on them for 3 whole hours.

My mate just kept buying this popcorn that he kept constantly eating while I slept for about an hour and a half. When I woke up, there were some guys sitting beside us. I asked one guy if the competition has started and he replied, "Sleep. Plenty of time left" And thus I went back to sleep. It was tiring. I felt like I was in a battlefield waiting for commands and trying to survive. When I woke up by noon, I perceived people entering the building and guessed that the competition is due to start and went inside. I was quite anxious whether my left arm would tear while boxing, but I shook the anxiety off. It wasn't the time to worry. My match was set as the 9th and there was still 8 matches before me. I had plenty of time. While wearing my outfit, my stomach suddenly began to hurt. I wonder if the laxatives taking effect now?. The pain began to increase. I immediately went to the bathroom without a second thought. Why would these laxatives take effect at this moment before I compete? Just as I said, misfortune after misfortune. As if the whole world turned against us…

Once I had done my stretches and warm-up, I sat waiting for my match while watching the current ones. In one of them this guy lost by TKO in the 3rd round. I could see how he was in shock that he had lost. After stepping outside the ring, he began to tear up. I could see the pain in his expression. I couldn't just see it but feel it. Everything ending in mere seconds after all the hard work he had put in. I felt for the guy, but it is what it is. He had to keep moving forward…

When I heard my name called out, I went to the red corner and stepped inside the ring. I was ready and confident, but I had no second beside me. I was all alone. It hadn't mattered for me. I was fine being alone. I ended up winning by TKO in the first round. I knew it would end soon for, after the first punch, I realised my hand hurt him. I pounded him a couple of times, and the referee called in for a stop. I did not even feel like I competed after stepping out of the ring. Some of my friends I've made throughout my competitions came to greet me afterwards. I felt great. I packed my things and returned to the hotel afterwards.

"It is about a quarter to ten whilst writing these notes at the moment. I've only eaten a half a can of tuna. I would need to weigh in tomorrow yet again. I don't feel starvation as much for the joy of winning is distracting the pain. We're having a good atmosphere at the moment. At least part of the distress is gone. My mate is set to compete tomorrow. He had taken a laxative to make sure he makes his weight. Hope all goes well."

19TH OF NOVEMBER
WEIGH-IN DAY

Whilst sleeping today, I heard my friend jumping out of bed and going to the bathroom for about 15 minutes. Once he got out, he kept complaining about how his stomach hurts. The laxatives had done their work.

We have woken up and arrived at our destination just as yesterday. We performed the same course of action while weighing in. After we were done with this bloody weigh-in, we walked to the side of the building at the place where the chairs were located. We stayed there until the competition time, which was 3 hours from now. Today, instead of popcorn, he kept buying noodles. I slept throughout the 3 hours. When I woke up after my nap, it was about noon.

I looked towards my mate, and I realised he was nervous. It was his first competition, so it was understandable. I tried to comfort him while he was wearing his outfit. I kept telling him to dictate the match. To push with his left. His match was set to be the 11th. When he stepped inside the ring, I observed how his hands were quite shaky. I cried, "don't lose control." I hoped it would help him. Unfortunately, he ended up losing by points. He did a great job in his first competition. Did his best. He gave it all he had. There was nothing he could do. I kept cheering him during the match, but he told me his hearing was completely shut off. I comforted him after the match for I saw how disappointed he was. I tried my best to make him feel better. I hope I fulfilled that. I didn't have a match today, so we left for our hotel.

"It's now 11:00 PM. The atmosphere isn't as cheerful. After returning from the competition, my mate hadn't a reason to keep a diet anymore so he ate what he craved. He asked me if it was all right for me, and I replied with, "eat what you please." I knew food would make him feel better at least. My mate ate a shawarma sandwich, and I ate half a can of tuna with some blackberries while watching television. Once we ate, we took a nap. There wasn't much talking. My mate was quite down, and I needn't bother him. I took a 1-hour nap and got up at about 7:00 PM. There is no weigh-in tomorrow as it is a national holiday, but I was determined to train today and rest for tomorrow. Once I woke up from my nap, I went to a local garments store and bought some sportswear as I didn't have any sportswear to train with since I wasn't expecting the weigh-in to be every day. Regardless, once I was back in my room, I wore 3 layers on me. A first layer consisting of a normal shirt and undergarments, a second layer of trash bags, and a third and final layer of a hoodie and sweatpants. Afterwards, I went to the hotel gym and had one tiring training session. I ran for about 1-hour, skipped rope for about 10-minutes, and did some shadow boxing. I had no energy left in me to move anymore. I literally couldn't take my clothes off. I collapsed in the changing room. I lay on my back for about half an hour, staring at the ceiling. I had no more power to get up. At last, after my heart rate slightly decreased, I had enough power to take off my outfit and take a cold shower.

I hadn't even the energy to pack my garments up so I just left them at the gym, that I wouldn't need anymore.

"I just came from the hotel's gym and I have no energy in me. My mate just woke up from his nap. His expression conveys that he is feeling better at least. I have no more energy in me to continue writing so I only wrote what is important. I don't know for how long I can last in this state. My mouth is thirsty, my lips are so dry that they bleed if I open my mouth too wide, and my hallucinations about food is coming back. I have been dehydrated for some days now. I don't know even know the reason why I'm fighting anymore."

20TH OF NOVEMBER

124.5LBS (56.5KGS)

Nothing special had occurred on the 20th. My weight was as I wanted it to be. My mate was feeling better. Therefore, the atmosphere in the air relaxed. I hadn't trained. I solely relaxed. I've only needed to distract myself from thinking about water. I was dehydrated for a couple of days. My body needed water. I spent the whole day watching food clips and television channels. I felt like I was having a slow demise. I remember absolutely nothing from the day. All I remember is me vaguely staring at the ceiling. All I seem to remember is the suffering…

"10:00 PM… All this suffering. All this hard work. Why am I suffering so much? I need some water. I don't even have saliva in my throat anymore. My face looks like a tomato dried from its juice. I want to end this suffering. I'm standing on thin glass. I hope it won't crack…"

21TH OF NOVEMBER

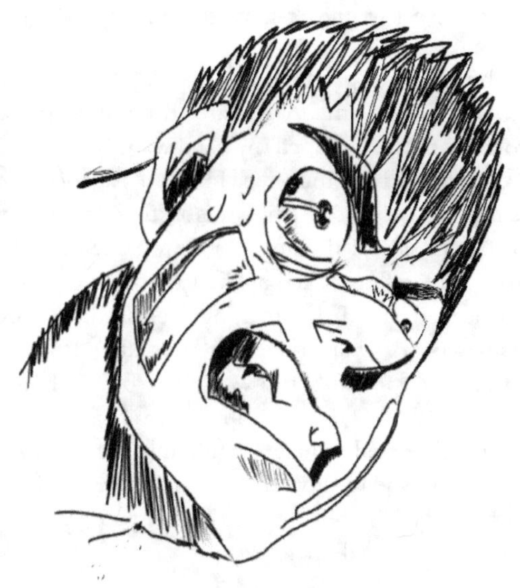

21TH OF NOVEMBER

WEIGH-IN DAY

woke up on that day in much distress. I still remember some of the hallucinations I had while sleeping that night. We got up at 7:30 AM as you have come to know. I hadn't the energy to drive so we ordered a car to get us there. We arrived at about 9:00 AM. The official weigh-in had started. After weighing in, we waited at our normal spot where the chairs were. I had to have something to eat, or else I wouldn't have the energy to fight.

Thus, I ate a pack of biscuits and a protein bar. I took a nap untill noon time. Afterwards, I began to prepare myself. I wore my outfit, wrapped my hand wraps around, and did some stretching and warming up. It was a patience game now. My match was set as the 7th. I was in the red corner, so I stayed close to its side of the ring. Once my name was called, I stepped inside. The referee asked if I had a second, I declined. He asked if I needed one, I declined, but he asked for someone to act as my second. Once the match had started, I knew I was more elite. My opponent's footwork was off. I threw my leading hand, and he suddenly jumped forward towards me with his body and started punching randomly. I could see his punches clearly, but when I slipped through one, he would push my head downwards. The referee then would pause the match and ask me to lift my head up.

At first, I approved, but when it became repetitive, I began to protest. He wasn't accepting any of my protests. At one point the guy was clearly holding my hands, and I thus circled the guy to let go of my hands. The referee called it a fault upon me and asked the judges to deduct 1 point from ME. I was in complete disbelief. "What was happening right now?" I thought at the time. The guy was clearly making the faults. He was a complete brawler. I was boxing. In the interval between the second and third round, my second advised me that if I wanted to win, I would need to knock the guy out. I despaired. I forgot my boxing. The bloody guy kept running away, and once we were clutching, he would rabbit punch me. The referee wouldn't say a word. My protests weren't getting at him. I... I don't know what was happening. I still get outraged when I recall those moments. I snapped. The devil got inside of me. I lost my control. All the misfortunes that have been happening to us. I couldn't keep it in anymore.

I completely lost control. I kept pushing to get at him, and I did get him a couple of times. At one moment he led with a left jab. I slipped through it, but he punched me in the back of my head. My head bent down due to the punch. I was just beginning to twist my hip to come up with a left hook when I find the referee pausing the game again. I stood completely still. "What?" "This referee… What is he doing."? I found him holding our hands and leading us to the middle of the ring. I knew what was coming. I bloody knew. The referee raised the arm of the guy and ruled it a win by TKO for him.

It feels like a dream. I did not actually get what happened at the time except when I got out of the building. I did not want to believe what had occurred. Once I stepped out of the ring, I packed my things and got out. Before I got out of the building, two guys from the national team asked me what I had done. I told them that I've lost by TKO.

They replied by saying that they don't know what the referee was doing. That the guy kept pushing my head downwards and I had the upper hand most of the time. Once I got out of the building, it all came back to me. I remembered the match in mere seconds through my head. I realised it was futile now, my journey had ended. After all the hard work I put in this, the stress, the training, and the starvation; it came to an end in an instant. I kept holding on to the pain for so long and it all ended with the hands of this referee. I held on to the frustration and pain for so long, but I couldn't keep it in anymore. I let go of my bag and collapsed on to the ground crying. I let it all out. All the pain. All the hard work. The tears helped me get on with what I had faced.

I cried and cried. Disbelief. Pain. "What should I do now?" "How would I face my father?" "What should I tell him?" These questions kept coming back and forth at the time. My mate tried to cheer me up, but he seemed in disbelief alongside me. He had faith in me. I told him that I would get a gold medal. That I would come first. That I would allow him to see me as one of the best. I was embarrassed. I couldn't fulfill my promises. I wanted to apologise but I couldn't. Why were these misfortunes occurring?

During the drive back to the hotel, the atmosphere was silent and clenched. Ultimately this was the end of our journey. We returned back to our city after returning to the hotel and packing our belongings.

"It is 10:00 PM. I'm writing this from my home. We returned from our journey. My journey has ended. I can't endure the aching inside my chest. I'm having teary eyes at the moment. I lost my match during the quarterfinals. I'm not going to whine around about my loss. I take my losses like a man. But it felt like a conspiracy against me rather than a match.

I am hurt. Deeply… After all the hard work I've put and all this starvation. I am completely confident that I have worked the hardest amongst these players. I've had the strictest diet for a month. And it just ended… The hardest part was facing my father. After giving him the news, he told me "It's okay. Relax for a couple of days and focus on what is important now." He hasn't got a clue what's inside my chest at the moment. I couldn't get my father to respect my dreams. To respect my decisions. To acknowledge me. I wanted to make him proud. I wanted to show him that I can become successful too. I wish I could tell him, "I have done it." I haven't done it… I couldn't make him acknowledge me. It doesn't even matter anymore. Today, I have been wounded deeply."

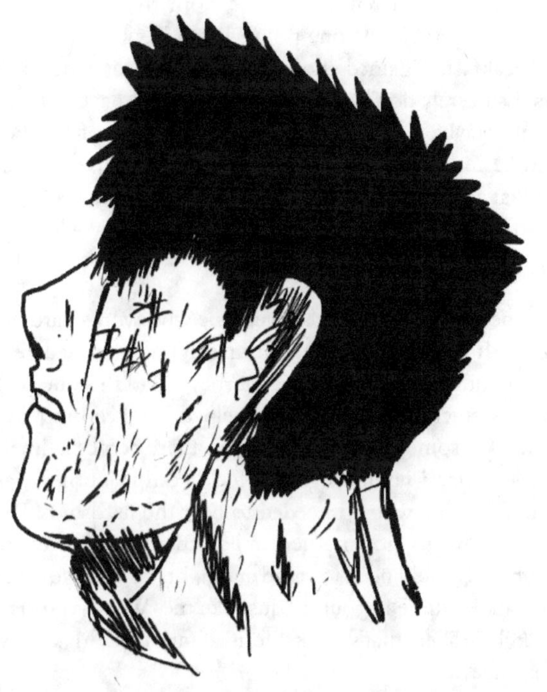

POSTFACE:

It was a long journey. There has been much suffering throughout this journey. I can't describe the suffering in words. As if a part of me had been taken away and will never return. All the running I did when everyone else was sleeping. I can't seem to forget how I started with hunger, which led to starvation and eventually to thirstiness. The wound hasn't healed until today.

Making my father proud… I wanted him to acknowledge me. The pain seemed too real at the time. Regardless of what had happened, when I returned home from the competition. My diet was miserable. At one point, I was having chocolate bars for breakfast. I gained those 25 pounds I lost back in mere days. I sincerely don't know the reason why I have written such a book. Maybe to get the distress I have felt out of me. Perhaps to share my experience. Perhaps to show people that weight isn't lost as easily as some people think. If more people put in the effort to lose even 1 pound, I am sure they would be proud of themselves…

At the end of the day, not everyone who works hard gets rewarded. It is what it is. I won't survive in the jungle if I get stuck in the middle. Throughout this journey, I had this one sentence that was stuck in my head that helped me keep moving forward… "at some stage in a man's life, there comes a time when he has to stand up and fight." I feel like this journey was one stage of my life where I needed to bear the hardships. Perhaps I would come to face another similar situation in my upcoming life where I would need to stand and fight. Perhaps you will face a demanding time in your life just like me. Would you stand up and fight? Then that's what life is all about… Make it worth your while…

SUPPORT THE AUTHOR:

I self-publish privately. therefore, anyone, if interested, can support me and check out my services on my website:

www.amirjoy.net

PICTURE CREDITS:

All pictures and images are supplied and illustrated by the author.

—

www.ingramcontent.com/pod-product-compliance
Lightning Source LLC
Chambersburg PA
CBHW061506250726
48657CB00005B/1739